144 HERBAL REMEDIES TO KNOW BEFORE 2024

Eliyah Mashiach

Disclaimer

The information provided in this book by Eliyah Mashiach is for general informational purposes.

UNDER NO CIRCUMSTANCES SHALL WE BE LIABLE TO YOU FOR ANY LOSS OR DAMAGE OF ANY KIND INCURRED AS A RESULT OF YOUR USE OF THE SITE, OR DEPENDENCE ON ANY INFORMATION CONTAINED ON THIS SITE, OR USE OF ANY INFORMATION CONTAINED ON THIS SITE OR BOOK. USING THE INFORMATION PROVIDED IS SOLELY AT YOUR OWN RISK.

CONTENTS

Introduction 5

Remedies For Acid Reflux 6

Remedies For Anemia 8

Remedies For Diabetes 10

Remedies For Bloating/Gastroenteritis 12

Remedies For Insomnia/Sleeping Disorders 13

Remedies For Eyes 15

Remedies For The Kidneys 17

Remedies for Arthritis 19

Remedies For Skin Care 21

Remedies For Migraines/Headaches 24

Remedies For Anxiety and Depression 26

Remedies For Yeast Infection 28

Remedies For Herpes & Cold Sores 30

Remedies For Nerve Repair 32

Remedies For The Heart 34

Remedies For Fever 35

Remedies For U.T.I 37

Remedies For Constipation 39

Remedies For Prostatitis...41

Remedies For Bad Breath..42

Remedies For Burns 43

Remedies For Diarrhea...45

Remedies For Allergies & Food Poisoning 47

Remedies For Toothache 49

Remedies For Earache..51

Remedies For High Blood Pressure 53

Remedies For ADHD 55

Conclusion..57

Introduction

Greetings everyone!!! I am Eliyah Mashiach a Natural Herbalist. In this book, I will be sharing with you all 144 herbal remedies that will benefit the entire family as well as your neighbors. I truly hope that you will find each remedy beneficial to the area/s that you need.

Remedies For Acid Reflux

For persons suffering from

Heartburn, Indigestion, Gastritis, GERD, H.Pylori, and Ulcers, here are some remedies you can use.

Remedy 1

1/4 cabbage

1/2 papaya

2 cups of water

Blend together strain and drink

Remedy 2

1\4 cup of cabbage

1 & 1/2 cups of water

Blend together strain and drink

Remedy 3

1/4 of cabbage

1 tablespoon ginger

2 cups of water

Blend together strain and drink

Remedy 4

1 teaspoon chamomile

1 cup hot water

Steep for 10 mins strain and drink

Remedy 5

1 teaspoon slippery elm

1 cup hot water

Steep for 10 mins strain and drink

Remedy 6

1 tablespoon grated ginger

2 cups hot water

Steep for 10 mins strain and drink

NB: Ripe papaya, papaya seeds, carrot, and almond milk can relieve acid reflux, heartburn, indigestion, etc.

Remedies For Anemia

For persons suffering from Iron

Deficiency, Low Blood Count, Fainting Spells, and Dizziness, and for women with Anemia due to heavy menstrual flow, here are some remedies to help.

Remedy 1

1 cup almond milk

1/4lb grapes

2 medium size beetroots

3 medium carrots

2 tablespoon honey

Blend beetroot and carrot in two cups of water then strain and add this juice to almond milk and grapes. Blend all ingredients together. Finally, strain (optional) and drink 2 cups per day.

NB: It is important for you to take in your vegetables and organic fruits.

Remedy 2

1 teaspoon stinging nettle

1 cup of hot water

Steep for 10 mins, strain and drink

Remedy 3

1/2 teaspoon gentian root

1 cup hot water

Steep for 10 mins, strain and drink

Remedy 4

Boil in 2 cups of water 1 cup of chopped, young green bananas for 10 mins. Allow cooling then strain. Use the water that is strained from the young bananas to blend 1 cup of callaloo, strain, and drink 1/4 of a cup in the morning and the same at night.

Remedies For Diabetes

For persons suffering from Diabetes, here are some natural remedies to help lower high blood sugar.

Remedy 1

Boil in 5 liters of water 15 mango leaves

20 cinnamon leaves

2 cups cerasee/bitter melon leaves 1 head of garlic. Boil for 10-15 mins. Store in refrigerator.

Drink 1 cup in the morning and the same at night.

Remedy 2

Boil in 4 cups of water 3 cinnamon leaves or 1 teaspoon of cinnamon powder, and 1 tablespoon of ginger. Drink 2 cups a day.

Remedy 3

Blend together in 2 cups of water

2 okras

1/2 of a cucumber

1/2 lime

1 teaspoon moringa leaves powder.

Strain and drink throughout the day.

Remedy 4

Boil in 4-6 cups of water 1 sprig of basil 1 sprig of neem leaves. Boil for 10 mins.

Drink 2 cups a day.

Remedy 5

Get unripe papaya, remove seeds, grate the fruit and use the poultice and apply to diabetic wounds.

Cover the poultice on the wound for 24 hours then change thereafter.

Remedies For Bloating/Gastroenteritis

For persons suffering from Bloating, or Gas, here are some remedies you can use.

Remedy 1

Boil in 2 cups of water for 10 mins, 1 tablespoon of grated ginger. Drink 1-2 cups each day.

Remedy 2

Add 1 teaspoon of activated charcoal to 1 cup of warm water. Drink 1- 3 cups a day.

Remedy 3

Steep in 2 cups of hot water for 10 mins, 1 sprig of lemon balm. Drink 2 cups a day.

Remedy 4

Steep in 2 cups of hot water for 10 mins, 1 sprig of peppermint. Drink 2 cups a day.

Remedies For Insomnia/Sleeping Disorders

For persons having difficulty sleeping here are some remedies that will help.

Remedy 1

Mix into 1 container equal parts of Ashwagandha, Blue Vervain, Chamomile, and St. John's Wort. Add 1 teaspoon of mixture to 1 cup of hot water. Strain and drink 1 cup before bed.

Remedy 2

Boil in 4 cups of water 3 soursop leaves. Boil for 7- 10 mins. Strain and drink 1 cup 2 times daily.

Remedy 3

Steep in 1 cup of hot water for 10 mins, 1 teaspoon of passion flower. Strain and drink 1 cup before bed.

Remedy 4

Boil in 2-4 cups of water for 7-10 mins, 1 sprig lemon balm, 1 sprig rosemary. Strain and drink 2 cups a day.

Remedy 5

Steep in 1 cup hot water for 10 mins, 1 teaspoon lavender. Strain and drink before bed.

Remedy 6

Steep in 2 cups of hot water for 10 mins, 1 teaspoon of skullcap, and 1 teaspoon of chamomile. Strain and drink 1 cup before bed.

Remedies For Eyes

For persons suffering from Dry Eyes, Glaucoma, Cataracts, and other Eye Related problems, here are some remedies you can use.

Remedy 1

1 handful of freshly reaped marijuana leaves. Wash leaves properly, and place them in cheesecloth.

Use a clean object to beat then squeeze the juice into a sterile container. Store in the refrigerator.

Drop 1-2 drops in both eyes morning and evening.

Remedy 2

Mix 1/2 teaspoon sea salt with 1 cup of room temperature water. Use 2 drops of the mixture in the eyes. Do this 2-3 times per day This remedy is excellent for conjunctivitis/pink eye.

Remedy 3

Blend 1/2 of a medium aloe vera leaf

Ground 1lb walnuts

1 & 1/3 cups organic honey

Freshly squeezed juice from four lemons Combine all ingredients and mix well.

Store in the refrigerator.

Take 1 tablespoonful three times per day. 30 minutes before breakfast, lunch, and dinner.

Take 2 weeks break between monthly treatments.

Remedy 4

Steep in 2 cups of hot water for 10 minutes, 1 teaspoon of eyebright, and 1 teaspoon of chamomile. Strain and drink 2 cups a day.

NB: Cold cucumbers can be placed over the eyes to relieve soreness. Eat a lot of berries!!!

Remedies For The Kidneys

For those who are suffering from kidney problems or kidney disease, or if you want to prevent kidney problems here are some remedies to use.

Remedy 1

1 whole beetroot

1 purple onion

1 tablespoon ginger

2 cloves garlic

2 cups of water

Blend all ingredients together

Strain and drink 2 times per day.

Remedy 2

Mix 1 teaspoon of dandelion in 1 cup of hot water.

Drink 2-3 times per day for one month.

Remedy 3

Boil in 4 cups of water for 10 mins, 1 handful of cornsilk. Drink throughout the day. Do this for 7 days.

Remedy 4

6 tablespoons pumpkin seed

1 teaspoon dandelion

1/2 teaspoon cinnamon powder

1 teaspoon honey

2 cups water

Blend all ingredients together and drink as often as desired.

NB: It is important to consume fresh organic fruits and vegetables.

Remedies for Arthritis

For those who are suffering from Joint Pains, Joint Inflammation, Rheumatism, and Circulatory problems, here are some remedies for you.

Remedy 1

Crush/blend 3 turmeric root

10 custard apple leaves 1/4 cup water or vinegar

Apply to the affected area.

Remedy 2

Boil in 2 cups of water for 10 mins, 1 tablespoon turmeric root, 1 tablespoon ginger root. Strain and drink 2 cups a day for up to a month then break.

Remedy 3

Boil in 4 cups water for 10 mins, 1 teaspoon devil's claw, 1 sprig rosemary 1 teaspoon organic turmeric powder. Strain and drink 2 cups a day.

Remedy 4

Infuse 1 cup of fresh rosemary in 2/3 cup olive oil.

Store in a dark area for 3 weeks. Use to massage affected areas.

Remedy 5

Add 1 teaspoon of cayenne pepper to 1 cup of room-temperature water. Mix and drink 3 times a day.

NB: Use ginger oil and cayenne pepper oil to massage inflamed joints to provide relief.

Remedies For Skin Care

Here are some remedies to help with

Skin Care, Skin Infections, Eczema, Insect Bites, Psoriasis, Acne, Boils etc.

Remedy 1

3 teaspoons neem

2 teaspoons ginger

4 teaspoons calendula/marigold

3 teaspoons turmeric

Combine all ingredients and use 1 heaping teaspoon to 1 cup of hot water

Let sit for 5 minutes then strain and drink 1 time per day.

Remedy 2

For skin detox, blend 1/4 cup aloe vera gel with 1 cup coconut water and drink. Do this remedy for 7 days.

Remedy 3

Boil in 1 gallon of water for 15 mins, 1/4lb neem leaves, and 1/4lb tamarind leaves. As warm as you can bear use it to bathe yourself.

This will help to treat hives, chicken pox, eczema, psoriasis, and other skin infections.

Remedy 4

Hot Infuse 1/4lb neem leaves in 1&1/2 cups of olive oil. Store in a dark place for 4-6 weeks. Apply to skin irritations, chafed skin, cracked lips, dry skin, psoriasis, acne, and other fungal infections.

Remedy 5

Burn 4 garlic cloves in 1/4 cup coconut oil. This should be done on low heat so that garlic is properly infused in coconut oil. Let cool and apply to dry flaky skin and scalp. This can also be applied to other fungal and skin infections. This remedy can be applied as often as needed.

Remedy 6

Blend in 1 cup of coconut water, 1/2 of a cucumber.

This will hydrate and allow the skin to glow. Drink 2 cups a day.

NB: It is very important for you to cut back significantly on fatty, greasy foods and sodas. Incorporate more fresh organic fruits and vegetables into your diet.

Remedies For Migraines/Headaches

For persons having Migraines and Headaches here are some remedies, you can use.

Remedy 1

One of the simplest remedies of them all is to drink pure water and keep your body hydrated. Drink 6- 8 glasses of spring water a day along with consuming organic fruits and natural juices.

Remedy 2

Use 1-2 drops of lavender oil on the temples. This can be repeated 2-3 times a day.

Remedy 3

Boil in 2-4 cups of water for 10 mins, 3 bay leaves, and 1 tablespoon of ginger. Strain and drink 2-3 cups a day or when needed.

Remedy 4

Steep in 1 cup of hot water for 10 mins, 1 teaspoon of passion flower. Strain and drink when needed.

Remedy 5

Boil in 2-4 cups of water for 10 mins, 1 sprig of rosemary, and 3 soursop leaves. Strain and drink when necessary.

Remedy 6

Soak feet in warm water for 20 mins. After doing this massage your feet with rosemary oil. Repeat this as often as needed.

Remedy 7

Steep in 4 cups of hot water for 10 mins, 1 teaspoon blue vervain, 1 teaspoon skullcap, and 1 sprig of lemon balm. Strain and drink 2 cups a day or when needed.

Remedies For Anxiety and Depression

Here are some remedies for persons suffering from Anxiety and Depression.

Remedy 1

Steep in 1 cup of hot water for 10 mins, 1 teaspoon of passion flower. Strain and drink 2 cups a day.

Remedy 2

Boil in 2-4 cups of water for 10 mins, 1 sprig basil, and 1 sprig rosemary. Strain and drink 2 cups a day.

Remedy 3

Add calming essential oils to a diffuser for aromatherapy. Use oils such as lavender, eucalyptus, valerian, lemon balm, and peppermint. Do this, especially at night or when trying to relax.

Remedy 4

Steep in 2 cups of hot water for 10 mins, 1 teaspoon chamomile, and 1 teaspoon skullcap. Strain and drink 2 cups a day.

Remedy 5

Steep in 1 cup of hot water for 10 mins, 1 teaspoon St. John's Wort. Strain and drink 2 times a day.

Remedy 6

Combine together equal parts of all the dry herbs listed under anxiety and depression into one container. Take 1 teaspoon of mixed herbs and steep in 1 cup of hot water for 10 mins. Strain and drink 2 cups a day.

Remedies For Yeast Infection

For persons suffering from Yeast Infection here are some remedies you can use.

Remedy 1

Steep in 1 cup of hot water for 10 mins, 1 teaspoon of calendula/marigold. Drink 3 cup servings throughout the day for up to 7 days.

Remedy 2

Boil in 3 cups of water for 10 mins, 4 crushed garlic cloves. Drink 2 cups daily.

Remedy 3

Steep in 1 cup of hot water for 10 mins, ½ teaspoon golden seal. Strain and drink in two separate servings throughout the day.

Remedy 4

Boil in 6 cups of water for 10 mins, 1 cup of oregano, 4 cloves of garlic, 1 teaspoon of dandelion, and 3 teaspoons of calendula. Strain and store in the refrigerator. Drink 1 cup a day.

Remedy 5

Soak overnight in 2 cups coconut water, 4 chopped okras, and 2 chopped garlic cloves. Drink 2 cups a day for up to 1 month then break.

NB: Infusion(s) made from garlic, golden seal, and calendula when properly strained can be used for douching.

Remedies For Herpes & Cold Sores

For those suffering from Herpes, there are herbs that can help you to prevent an outbreak and also help to alleviate symptoms during an outbreak.

Remedy 1

Mix equal parts of these herbs into 1 container. St. John's Wort, chamomile, lemon balm, bladderwrack, and dandelion. Steep in 1 cup of hot water for 10 mins, 1 teaspoon of this mixture of herbs. Strain and drink 2 cups a day.

Remedy 2

Boil in 6 cups of water 1 sprig of lemon balm, 1 sprig of rosemary, 3 oregano leaves and 3 teaspoons of calendula. Strain and refrigerate. Drink 1 -2 cups a day.

Remedy 3

Steep in 2 cups of hot water for 10 minutes, 1 teaspoon of chamomile and 1 tablespoon crushed ginger. Strain and drink when needed.

Remedy 4

For cold sores use tea tree oil, lemon balm oil, and oregano oil to help treat and heal blisters.

> **NB: It is important that changes be made in one's diet in order to see better results when taking herbs. Eat more organic fruits and vegetables. It is also important to get adequate rest.**

Remedies For Nerve Repair

For persons suffering from Pain as a result of Damaged Nerves or an Inflamed Nervous System.

Here are some remedies you can use.

Remedy 1

Get soursop fruit and eat it daily.

Remedy 2

Steep in 2 cups of hot water for 10 mins, 3 soursop leaves, and 1 teaspoon of St. John's Wort. Strain and drink 1 cup in the morning and 1 cup before bed.

Remedy 3

1 teaspoon of passion leaves

1 teaspoon basil

1 teaspoon rosemary

2 cups of boiling water

Place the 3 ingredients in the 2 cups of boiling water, and let steep for 5-10minutes Strain and drink before going to bed.

Remedy 4

1 sprig of lemon balm

2 soursop leaves

2 small stalks of chamomile /Spanish needle

1 tablespoon of turmeric

6 cups of hot water

Place all ingredients in boiling water, boil for 10 minutes. Strain, and store in the refrigerator. Drink 2 cups a day.

Remedies For The Heart

For those suffering from heart related problems and illnesses here are some remedies to help you.

Remedy 1

1 teaspoon Black cohosh

1 teaspoon cayenne pepper Mix all ingredients thoroughly. Use 1 heaping teaspoon to 1 cup of hot water. Steep for 10 minutes. Drink 2-3 cups a day, one in the morning and one before bed.

Remedy 2

Mix equal parts of angelica powder, hawthorn powder, and cayenne pepper in 1 container. Use 1 teaspoon to 1 cup hot water, and steep for 10 mins. Strain and drink 1-2 cups per day.

Remedy 3

Mix equal parts of black cohosh, goldenseal, and cayenne pepper into 1 container. Use 1 teaspoon to 1 cup of hot water. Steep for 10mins. Strain and drink 1-2 cups a day.

Remedy 4

Mix equal parts of lily of the valley, blue vervain, and cayenne pepper in 1 container. Use 1 teaspoon to 1 cup of hot water. Steep for 10 mins. Strain and drink 1-2 cups a day.

Remedies For Fever

For persons suffering from Fever, here are some remedies you can use.

Remedy 1

Steep in 2 cups of hot water for 10 mins, 1 tablespoon of grated ginger, and a pinch of cayenne pepper. Strain and drink 2-3 cups a day.

Remedy 2

Mix 1 teaspoon of cayenne pepper into 1 cup of warm water. Drink 1-3 cups a day

Remedy 3

Steep in 3 cups of hot water for 10 mins, 1 teaspoon chamomile, 1 teaspoon yarrow. Strain and drink 1- 3 cups a day.

Remedy 4

Boil in 4-6 cups of water for 10 mins, 1 tablespoon willow bark, and 1 tablespoon grated ginger. Strain and drink 1-3 cups a day.

Remedy 5

Boil in 4-6 cups of water for 10 mins, 4 chopped garlic cloves, 1 teaspoon cayenne pepper, and 1 tablespoon grated ginger. Strain and drink 1-3 cups a day.

Remedy 6

Blend in 1/4 cup of water 1 chopped onion. When done, strain and add 1/4 teaspoon of cayenne pepper, and 1 teaspoon of organic honey to onion juice. Take this mixture throughout the day using teaspoon servings.

NB: Apply cold sponge baths or warm sponge baths when necessary. Keep the person hydrated.

Remedies For U.T.I

For persons suffering from Urinary Tract Infections here are some remedies you can use.

Remedy 1

1 teaspoon dandelion root

1 teaspoon milk thistle

1 teaspoon licorice

1 teaspoon borotutu

Combine all ingredients and use 1 heaping teaspoon to 1 cup of hot water. Steep for 10 mins, strain and drink 1-2 cups a day.

Remedy 2

Steep in 2 cups of hot water for 10 mins, 1 handful of cornsilk, and 2 chopped garlic cloves. Strain and drink 2 cups a day for 7 days.

Remedy 3

Steep in 3 cups of hot water for 10 mins, 1 teaspoon of uva-ursi leaves, and 1 teaspoon of dandelion root. Strain and drink 2-3 cups a day.

Remedy 4

Steep in 4 cups hot water for 10 mins, 1 sprig peppermint, 1 sprig rosemary, 1/2 teaspoon golden seal, and 1 teaspoon chamomile. Strain and drink 2 cups a day.

Remedy 5

Mix 1 tablespoon of apple cider vinegar in 250 ml of room temperature water. Drink 2 cups a day, for 7 days.

NB: Drinking organic cranberry juice will help with U.T.I. It is important for us to eat healthier and make better health choices.

Remedies For Constipation

For a person suffering from Constipation here are some remedies that you can use.

Remedy 1

Mix 1 tablespoon of grounded flax seeds in 1 cup of warm water. Drink 2 cups a day.

Remedy 2

Drink 1 cup of prune juice along with 1 teaspoon of olive oil in the mornings.

Remedy 3

Steep in 2 cups of hot water for 10 mins, 1 teaspoon of yellow dock. Strain and drink 12 cups a day.

Remedy 4

Mix 1/4 teaspoon cascara sagrada in 1/2 cup of warm water. Stir well and drink, first thing in the morning or just before bed.

Remedy 5

Steep for 10 mins 1/2 teaspoon of senna leaves powder in 1 cup of hot water. Strain and drink a cup serving 1-3 times a day.

Remedy 6

Blend in 1 & 1/2 cups of water 1 cup pineapple, and 1 cup cucumber. Do not strain. Drink 1 cup a day for 7 days.

Remedy 7

Soak overnight in 2 cups of coconut water, 4 chopped okras. Consume all the above portion throughout the day.

NB: It is very important to consume enough fibre, vegetables and fruits.

Remedies For Prostatitis

For persons suffering from Prostate problems here are some remedies to help you.

Remedy 1

Blend 3 & 1/2 tablespoons sunflower seeds, 3 & 1/2 tablespoons shelled pumpkin seeds, 3 & ½ tablespoon almond, and 1 teaspoon blue vervain in 1 & 1/2 cups water. Drink this throughout the day.

Remedy 2

Steep in 2 cups of hot water for 10 minutes, 1 teaspoon of saw palmetto, and 1 teaspoon of blue vervain. Strain and drink 1 cup in the morning after breakfast and 1 cup after supper.

Remedy 3

Steep for 10 mins, 1 teaspoon of gravel root in 1 cup of hot water. Strain and drink 1 cup before bed.

Remedy 4

Steep in 2 cups of hot water for 10 minutes, 1 teaspoon of stinging nettle root powder. Strain and drink 2 cups a day.

Remedy 5

Boil in 4 cups of water for 10 mins, 4 chopped garlic cloves and 1 tablespoon of grated ginger. Strain and drink 2 cups a day.

Remedies For Bad Breath

For those who are suffering from Bad Breath here are some remedies to help.

Remedy 1

Get freshly squeezed Spanish needle/chamomile leaf juice and use as a mouthwash. Use up to 3 times a day.

Remedy 2

Make tea using 1 sprig of peppermint to 1 cup of hot water. Steep for 10 mins. Add 2-3 drops of myrrh and use it as a mouthwash. Use throughout the day.

Remedy 3

Chew 1 Cardamom pod for about 5-10 mins after each meal. Do this as often as is needed.

Remedy 4

Steep in 2 cups of hot water for 10 mins, 1 teaspoon of fennel seeds. Strain and drink as needed.

Remedies For Burns

For all those who are suffering from different types of Burns, here are some remedies for you.

Remedy 1

1/4 cup of aloe vera,1/3 cup of water, 2 tablespoons of honey, and 9 tablespoons of turmeric powder.

Blend together and use on affected skin up to 3 times a day. Store in refrigerator.

Remedy 2

Use pure honey on wounds and scars for healing.

Honey can be applied up to 3 times a day on wounds.

Remedy 3

Apply aloe vera gel to the affected area 3 times a day.

Remedy 4

Steep in 4 cups of hot water for 10 mins, 1 sprig of rosemary, and 2 teaspoons chamomile. Strain and drink 2 cups a day.

Remedy 5

Juice fresh Spanish needle/chamomile and apply to the affected area 3 times a day.

Remedy 6

Steep in 1 cup of hot water for 10 mins, 1 teaspoon of stinging nettle. Drink 2 cups a day.

Remedy 7

Use poultice made from comfrey leaves, custard apple leaves, neem leaves, stinging nettle, or chamomile. Apply to affected areas.

Remedies For Diarrhea

For those suffering from Diarrhea and Irritable Bowel Syndrome. Here are some remedies that can help.

Remedy 1

Mix 1 teaspoon of activated charcoal in 1 cup of warm water. Drink 3 cups throughout the day.

Remedy 2

Steep in 1 cup of hot water for 10 minutes, 1 teaspoon of slippery elm powder. Strain and drink 1-3 cups a day.

Remedy 3

Steep in 4 cups of hot water for 10 mins, 1 tablespoon of chopped ginger, and 2 teaspoons of chamomile. Strain and drink 1-3 cups a day.

Remedy 4

Steep in 1 cup of hot water for 10 mins, 1 teaspoon of psyllium husk. Strain and drink 1-3 cups a day.

Remedy 5

Steep in 1 cup of hot water for 10 mins, 1 teaspoon of marshmallow powder. Strain and drink 1-3 cups a day.

Remedy 6

Steep in 4 cups of hot water for 10 mins, 1 sprig of peppermint, and 1 sprig of rosemary. Strain and drink 1-3 cups a day.

Remedies For Allergies & Food Poisoning

For those who are suffering from seasonal allergies and food poisoning, here are some remedies you can use.

Remedy 1

Boil in 3 cups of water, 1 tablespoon of Bizzy (Kola Acuminata) for 10 mins. Strain drink 1- 3 cups a day.

Remedy 2

Steep in 4 cups of hot water for 10 mins, 1 sprig of peppermint, and 1 sprig of rosemary. Strain and drink 1-3 cups a day

Remedy 3

Steep in 1 cup of hot water for 10 mins, 1 teaspoon of Mullein. Strain and drink 1-3 cups a day.

Remedy 4

Steep in 1 cup of hot water for 10 mins, 1 teaspoon of chamomile. Strain and drink 1-3 cups a day.

Remedy 5

Use diffusers for aromatherapy with these essential oils. Tea tree oil, Lemon balm oil, Peppermint oil, Eucalyptus oil, etc.

Remedy 6

Steep in 1 cup of hot water for 10 mins, 1 teaspoon of stinging nettle. Strain and drink 1-3 cups a day.

Remedies For Toothache

For persons suffering from Toothache or Pain from an Extracted Tooth, here are some remedies you can use.

Remedy 1

For a tooth just extracted bite down firmly on a green tea bag for 20-30 mins. This helps with blood clotting and pain relief. You can use a chamomile/peppermint tea bag.

Remedy 2

Apply 1-2 drops of clove oil to the affected tooth.

This can be done 2-3 times a day.

Remedy 3

Chew on a garlic clove near the affected tooth.

Remedy 4

Boil in 4 cups of water for 10 mins, 3 guava leaves, and 2 teaspoons of chamomile. Strain and use as a mouthwash.

Remedy 5

Boil in 2 cups of water for 10 mins, 3-4 cloves. Strain and use as a mouthwash. Use this 2-3 times a day.

Remedy 6

Mix 1/2 teaspoon sea salt in 1 cup of warm water. Use this mixture as a gargle 2-3 times a day.

Remedies For Earache

For a person suffering from Ear Pain and an Ear Infection, here are some remedies that you can use.

Remedy 1

Make garlic oil using 4 chopped garlic cloves hot infused in 4 tablespoons of olive oil. Use 1-2 drops on the cotton ball and place the cotton ball in the affected ear.

Remedy 2

Apply a warm chamomile tea bag or poultice to the affected ear. Do this up to 3 times a day.

Remedy 3

Apply warm thyme or rosemary oil around the affected ear lobe. Do this 3 times a day.

Remedy 4

Boil in 4 cups of water for 10 mins, 4 chopped garlic cloves, and 3 oregano leaves. Strain and drink 1 cup 3 times a day.

Remedy 5

Apply warm ginger oil around the affected ear. This can be done 1-3 times a day.

Remedy 6

Mix 1/4 teaspoon of golden seal powder with 1 cup of water or juice. This can be done 2-3 times per day.

Remedy 7

Boil in 4 cups of water for 10 mins, 1 sprig thyme, and 1 sprig rosemary. Strain and drink 1-3 cups a day.

Remedies For High Blood Pressure

For all those suffering from High Blood pressure, here are some remedies that you can use.

Remedy 1

Boil in 5 liters of water 15 mango leaves, 1 heaping handful of cerasee (bitter melon), 20 cinnamon leaves, and 1 head of garlic.

Strain, refrigerate, and drink 2 cups a day.

Remedy 2

Boil in 4 cups of water for 10 mins, 4 chopped garlic cloves. Strain and drink 2 cups a day.

Remedy 3

Steep in 3 cups of hot water for 10 mins, 1 tablespoon grated ginger, and 3 cinnamon leaves. Strain and drink 1-3 cups a day.

Remedy 4

Steep in 4 cups of hot water for 10 mins, 1 sprig of basil, and 1 tablespoon of grated ginger. Strain and drink 1-3 cups a day.

Remedy 5

Steep in 1 cup of hot water for 10 mins, ½ teaspoon of Ginkgo Biloba. Drink 2 cups a day.

Remedy 6

Steep in 4 cups of hot water for 10 minutes, 1 sprig of thyme, 2 teaspoons of chamomile, and 1 teaspoon of grated ginger. Strain and drink 1-3 cups a day.

Remedies For ADHD

For all those who are suffering from Attention Deficit Hyperactivity Disorder, here are some remedies that will help you.

Remedy 1

Steep in 1 cup of hot water for 10 mins, 1 teaspoon of chamomile. Strain and drink 1-2 cups a day.

Remedy 2

Steep in 1 cup of hot water for 10 mins, ½ teaspoon of Ginkgo Biloba. Strain and drink 1-2 cups a day.

Remedy 3

Boil in 4 cups of water for 10 mins, 1 sprig of rosemary, and 1 sprig of peppermint. Strain and drink 1-3 cups a day.

Remedy 4

Steep in 2 cups of hot water for 10 mins, 1 sprig of lemon balm. Strain and drink 2 cups a day.

Remedy 5

Steep in 2 cups of hot water for 10 mins, 1 teaspoon of passionflower. Strain and drink 1-2 cups a day.

NB: It is important for persons with ADHD to avoid sugary foods. Make a change to your diet by adding more natural foods, juices, drinks, and smoothies. As much as possible avoid artificially processed foods.

Conclusion

144 Herbal Remedies To Know Before 2024, is a book designed to help guide you in using simple natural remedies to treat illnesses and alleviate their symptoms. We hope that as you read, you will benefit greatly from the general knowledge shared in this book.

We have more books on the way and we ask for your continuous support as we bring helpful and informative knowledge in this time of **climatic changes**. May our heavenly father Yahweh Elohiym and our savior Yahshua Ha Mashiach guide you on this journey to long life.

Please check our online herbal store at eliyahmashiachherbalstore.com or contact us by email at eliyahmachiach@gmail.com

Thank you for all the support and love family.

Made in United States
Troutdale, OR
11/12/2024

24723823R00033